SUSPICION *of* MALIGNANCY

DELORES BURGESS

UNITED
WRITERS PRESS, INC

United Writers Press, Inc.
P. O. Box 326
Tucker, Georgia 30085
1-866-857-4678

ISBN: 0-9760824-7-0
ISBN-13: 978-0-9760824-7-7

Library of Congress Control Number: 2005937321

Printed in the United States of America.
King Printing, Lowell, Massachusetts

Cover Design by Jeff Rogers, B.RogersMusic & Creative Services
Cover Photography: Carol Roach, PhotoOne/VideoOne
Performance Cameo (back cover): Johnnetta Fielder-Pitts,
    Awesome Effects Photography

I dedicate this book to every person God has allowed me to touch not only through infirmity, but also through the offerings of love, faith, inspiration, and hope.

Cover to cover, I dedicate the message of wellness, health, and care to the memory of my step-father, Eugene Cochran, who died of throat cancer on July 17, 2005.

And finally,
To Mrs. Gloria Brown,
a sweet holy filled prayer warrior, fighter, and breast cancer survivor who lost her husband just as she was transitioning in her cancer treatment from chemo to radiation. Mr. Marvin was a jolly fellow who loved laughter and enjoyed people and he will be sorely missed. Ms. Gloria, I hope the light of this book shines brightly on your already beaming personality and beautiful spirit. I'm glad I had a chance to spend time with you and Mr. Marvin together.

In Loving Memory of

Carolyn Merchant
Linda Radney
Donna Fields
Cassandra Benson
Sharazon Walters
Shabrina Williams
Ruthie Odum
Mitzi Mayes

Table of Contents

Acknowledgments

I could not have completed this project if it were not for the love and support of my husband, Gary Burgess and the patience of my children, Tiffany and Camaren. My motivation in the fight for life! Without them there would be no story. Thank you, honey, and sweet babies, for giving up your individual time with me while I pecked away at the computer vowing daily: "I'm almost done!"

My mother, Lillie Cochran, deserves a mighty hand for her strength and unfailing tenacity to see me through my infirmity when she had her own. Her example fueled my determination to get up and not feel sorry for myself. I thank my brother, Roger, for introducing me to the blessings of the book, "Purpose Driven Life." He had no idea how on time his witness to the book's impact on his life was for me—perfect—right when I could have lost my mind! I acknowledge all of my siblings, in-laws, nieces, nephews, cousins, aunts and uncles for their prayers and words of encouragement along the way. They brought Christmas 2003 to me in Atlanta while I was in recovery.

I thank my influences, mentors, spiritual leaders, motivators, friends, and fans for their love, prayers, and encouraging anticipation of my next CD. Your prayers for my healing and deliverance have made that possible. I hope you are equally blessed by the book. I am so deeply honored to join my spiritual father, Pastor Gary Hawkins, Sr., as a published writer. He superbly taught me the substance of faith.

There are a host of individuals and organizations that have fed knowledge and understanding of breast cancer and the importance of support into my world. Clara Walton of Sisters Network-Atlanta Chapter, Dr. Rogsbert Phillips and Sisters By Choice, The American Cancer Society, The Georgia Cancer Foundation, Morehouse School of Medicine, Sandra Hamilton and Men Against Breast Cancer, The Witness Project, and the Centers for Disease Control and Prevention to name a few. Everything you offer is vital to the healing and wellness of cancer patients and their families. I thank you for all you do to promote and celebrate healthy living, life, and survivors.

My most gracious thanks go to the angels who helped edit my work so I could finally get this book into your hands. Vickie McGoy, Joyce Carr, Nynikka Palmer, Suzette Henry, June Reed, and Sandra Hamilton. Individually they are the best; collectively they are too much! Besides "Thank you" and "I love you," I'm out of words to express my gratitude and appreciation for how diligently they worked without hesitation, gripe, or slack. Draft after draft they made sure I pushed for the excellence and poignancy I wanted the book to convey. Their input, insight, and insults—okay constructive criticisms—stretched me to deliver the pit of my heart and soul onto every page. And to Vally Sharpe, my shero of editors. On-time and God-sent, she put my sometimes quirky expressions through the writer's wringer. Line for line she smoothed out the bumps and wrinkles leaving a smooth flow from which my voice could still be heard loud and clear.

Because of all of these guys, I can proudly say I have given my best!

Foreword

God's word clearly tells us that people perish for a lack of knowledge. We must learn to become knowledgeable in every area of our lives; especially our health. Our very nature causes us to procrastinate. However, behind the procrastination usually is the truth as to why we may continue to put off our health. These areas typically include fear, low priority, denial of family medical history, and unfortunately for some, lack of insurance. Delores Burgess allows you to see inside the depths of her heart and shares a motivating message that will light a fire under anyone frozen in these underlying areas.

Suspicion of Malignancy was written to demonstrate a walk of faith through the awesome testimony of Delores Burgess. It is apparent that God took Delores on a journey that He knew she could handle even though she didn't know it herself. During the early stages I'm sure Delores asked, "Why Me?" and God's response was "Why Not You?" He needed someone who would not become a steadfast victim but in the end become victorious. He needed a warrior! He needed Delores Burgess!

Even though this book is a testimony of a female and breast cancer, it prompted me to seek and discover that breast cancer is not a female disease. This remarkable book should be shared and read by both genders. I am now challenged to educate my wife, daughters, sisters, mother, and mother in-love. I am even more challenged to educate myself, my sons, and my brother.

The next time you see a pink ribbon or you are approached to give a donation to a breast cancer organization, please remember Delores Burgess's testimony and the inspiration she has so lovingly given to others!

Bishop Gary Hawkins, Sr.
Voices of Faith Ministries
Stone Mountain, Georgia

This book is about Delores Burgess's journey from normality to the variety of emotions triggered by the news of her diagnosis of breast cancer. *Suspicion of Malignancy* treats with the myriad of reactions; shock, bewilderment, fear, disbelief and even the testing of her faith.

Page after page takes you from the unsuccessful hope and prayer to hear the word "benign" through a regimen of physician appointments, surgery, and therapies, and finally, the declaration and celebration of survival.

As a physician, I believe in the relationship between faith and healing. Not only does Delores make the faith-healing connection, she summoned it to successfully navigate her journey from despair to recovery and beyond.

Others similarly diagnosed would do well to model Delores in her search for information and facts, the regimen of informed decisions, adoption of appropriate therapies and the summoning of her spiritual foundation.

Rogsbert F. Philips, M.D.

SUSPICION *of* MALIGNANCY

Introduction

On October 28, 2003, my life changed, irrevocably and without warning. A rising gospel artist in full-time ministry with a family I adored, I was stopped in my tracks by two simple words. Breast cancer. The idea of being diagnosed with this disease had never crossed my mind, but that day, I would embark on a roller-coaster journey that would take me to the depths of despair and the heights of intimacy with God.

One might ask how a woman of strong faith became depleted to such a lowly level of nothingness. Let me tell you…it was easy. Try being blind-sided, clobbered, and knocked off your feet by news that you have a life-threatening disease, and in my case, one that kills more African-American women than those of any other race. You might be a little dazed, too.

My faith would be tested over and over as I struggled to decide what to do and tried to find my spiritual balance. But it was not my faith that I lost…it was my focus. God had been there, preparing me even a full year before the diagnosis, and He was there, with me, even in the midst of my devastation.

Twelve days after I received the news, God's angels whispered the sweetest challenge in my ear:

"Delores, you may have ended up in this situation without notice or choice, but how you go through it and how you come out of it is very much your choice!"

This book is a testament to the choice I made. Though I didn't know I was writing a book at the time, I started it the day God's angels shook me and urged me to speak my heart to Him. I read the scripture imprinted on the cover of a little green journal: "O Lord, in the morning will I direct my prayer unto Thee and will look up." (Psalm 5:3)

The message was clear. All I needed to do was look up. And I did.

Perhaps you are standing in similar shoes to those in which I stood two years ago. Perhaps you are facing some form of infirmity or adversity that has left you unable to process even your next moment. If so, my sister/brother, please be encouraged! This book was written for no other purpose than to inspire, encourage, and empower you.

If you are in the midst of dealing with the infirmity of breast cancer, know that my wholehearted prayer is that you receive healing, walk in deliverance, and live in celebration of life. God sent me ahead of you to be tested in the fire, protected by the trust and security of his Word, and delivered me a stronger woman so I could come and tell you that it is time—time for you to start walking on your journey. You don't have to walk alone, but you must consciously walk in faith. I pray that as you read this, each word will speak power and authority into your weakness and victory into your battle. I pray that you will open your mind, body, and soul and receive the message of life God has for you in these pages.

I know you! You are beautiful! Your strength comes from the Lord! And you trust that He will never leave you nor forsake you. Nothing and nobody can take that away!

With that said, let me humbly ask that you walk with me as I retrace the steps of my own life-altering journey. I have tried to be as candid as possible about every detail of my experience to date—the good, the bad, and the glorious—as I talk about medical issues, my thoughts and feelings, and the struggle to keep my eyes on God. I pray that reading my story will lead you to discover, in your heart of hearts, the true meaning of trust and faith…and bring you closer to our Creator than ever before.

Let's walk!

Chapter 1
Breast What? The Devastating Diagnosis

"Oh God, please don't let it be cancer!" I cried in dire panic! My brain was all jumbled and my heart was banging against my chest. "Lord, I know you are not going to let these people tell me I have breast cancer?!?! I know you're not! After all of my work, sacrifice, obedience, and all that I do for you, surely you would not allow me, your faithful child, to suffer with cancer!"

That Thursday had started out pretty much as any day, and I was in my car on the way to work when my general surgeon's office called to ask when I could come in to discuss my biopsy results.

"Come in? Can't you give them to me over the phone?" I asked.

"No, ma'am," she replied.

"Why not? The radiologist who performed the biopsy said she would give me the results over the phone...whether the news was good or bad!"

"I'm sorry," the caller responded. "Can we schedule you on Tuesday?"

By this point, I knew that further verbal exchange was pointless. Our conversation ended with my scheduling what would be the third appointment since the mammogram, but there was no way I was going to wait another five days to find out if I had breast cancer. I would be loony by then!

Come in, she says. What wasn't she telling me? I had to find out so I decided I would call the radiologist when I got to my office and get the blasted results from her!

In the meantime, I was driving down the road, fumbling over my thoughts, one minute pleading and the next bargaining with God out loud, shouting as if He couldn't hear me! "What is this?" No way! No, it's not cancer!"

In the midst of my panic, I thought of how calm I had been after hearing one month before that the results from my very first mammogram had been deemed "suspicious of malignancy." At forty-one years old, I was healthy and had no concerns about breast cancer. I had no symptoms, no lump, no history, nothing! Breast cancer seemed inapplicable to me and I had only had the mammogram because it was time to get one based on my age. I was a little shocked, but didn't overreact. My response was to pray and thoroughly rebuke Satan in the name of Jesus!

My doctor had recommended two general surgeons: Dr. Love* who turned out not to be available for a month, and Dr. Mann. I made an appointment with Dr. Mann, and went on with life as normal.

When we met with him, Dr. Mann told my husband (Gary) and me that he didn't feel there was anything to worry about, that it was possible what we were seeing on the mammogram were simply small calcifications. He had recommended the biopsy "just to be sure."

But something had obviously changed, and the closer I got to my office the more I knew I was in trouble. The chaos and confusion in my head kept me calling to God, when suddenly, through the cloud of my tears, I noticed some beautiful pink and white trees along the highway sitting in a sea of perfectly manicured, emerald green grass. Each blade swayed in motion like ocean waves. I made a mental note of this wonder, settled myself, and then tried to refocus my eyes on the road.

---

* My doctors' names have been changed for the sake of privacy. I replaced them with the gifts I came to associate with them.

By the time I arrived at my office, my anxiety level was at an all time high. I walked over to my desk and before I could sit down, my phone rang. It was the radiologist.

"Have you spoken to Dr. Mann yet?" she asked.

"No," I told her, "but I suspect there's something wrong because I received a call from his office and the caller wouldn't tell me anything over the phone."

She was silent. Then I heard her take a deep breath (I held mine) and I could hear the words rising in her throat. I wanted so badly to stop them but I couldn't. "Yes, Delores, the malignancy is positive. It's definitely breast cancer."

WHAM!!! My heart exploded! IT HURT SO BAD! The pain choked me as I crossed my arms over my breasts to hold them close. I was dizzy. My imagination took off and I saw horrific images of me sick, suffering, and eventually dying! I saw my husband without me and craved the assurance that he would be able to raise our two girls alone. My entire being ached for my family. In my mind I had already left them…my beautiful girls…they needed their mother! My heart was broken!

Gary was in his office when I called for him to come to me. I was devastated! He tried to console me by holding me in his arms, but I broke away to grieve alone. My ability to reason was impaired and I paced back and forth in the hallway crying and talking to myself. Where was my God? I didn't deserve this! AAAAH…I was so disappointed with God! Never had I felt so betrayed, violated, or abandoned!

For about ten minutes, I sank into a pit of hopelessness and derangement, imagining my funeral. Then, something yanked me into reason. My spiritual reins took over and cautioned me to get control of myself…and the scripture 2 Corinthians 10:5 came to my mind, "Casting down imaginations and any high thing that exhalteth itself against the knowledge of God, bringing into captivity every thought to the obedience of Christ."

I closed my eyes and remembered who I was and to whom I belonged. I saw again those trees I had seen while in the car. It dawned on me that God, hearing my distress call, had given me a sign by gently turning my eyes towards those trees. They were His evidence that He had all power to sustain me in the midst of a dark season. After all, it was late October and the trees and grass were beautiful as in spring.

What a vivid revelation! Before I knew it I was blasting Satan and the cancer, "God has not given me a spirit of fear but one of power and of love and of a sound mind!" (2 Timothy 1:7). It is through Christ Jesus that I have the power and authority over all sickness and diseases. I have the power of FAITH!!! Whew! Thank God, my spirit was now aligned and ready for battle.

I can't say the same for my flesh, though. I WAS HURT! A complete emotional mess! I kept saying it over and over again: "Breast Cancer…a life threatening disease…ME… WOW?! I can't believe it! I absolutely cannot believe it!"

Fewer than fifteen minutes before I had been a vibrant, energetic individual conquering the challenges of a musical career and vying for my divine destiny in this life. That year, 2003, had been a phenomenal year for me! I was riding high on an award-winning season as a gospel recording artist, carving my mark in the industry, and making great ministerial strides. Music, television and radio appearances, travel, conferences, and business matters consumed my days. I was in supreme vocal shape and blessed with an itinerary that would keep me busy through the entire year. I had gracefully juggled my new career, my dedication to Gary and our two beautiful and talented daughters, and a heap of extracurricular activities. I had it all.

Then, in the blink of an eye, everything I lived for and aspired to accomplish seemed to have vanished.

I only wanted to please God and maintained a sincere desire to reach a higher level in Him. I had even asked Him to draw me closer and deeper into intimacy with Him. My girlfriend, Suz, had always told me, "Girl, you better be careful what you pray for! You don't know what you may have to go through to get it," but I had never expected Him to use breast cancer to answer my prayer.

Finally I asked myself, "What now, Delores? All things in perspective, God has cast His will." (This was no trick of the devil although I'm sure he enjoyed my moment of insanity and would have preferred it to last a lot longer.) My situation was clearly a matter between God and me. Like it or not, we had an agreement. He had control over my life. My job was to trust Him and act according to His plan, His will, and His way—not mine.

Nevertheless, I was not bound to claim breast cancer as mine, give in to it, or take ownership of it. A firm believer that we become what we perceive ourselves to be, I wasn't about to become breast cancer and breast cancer was not about to become me. If we see or claim victory we'll be victorious!

Giving in was not an option for me. I decided to trust God and let Him guide me through the process.

Chapter 2
Who Said I Was Having Surgery?

The days ahead were humbling, hurtful, and frightening. Ten singing engagements remained on my calendar and despite this news, I was determined to keep every commitment; God's grace would have to hold me up. Coping became an out of body experience. I was still quite numb yet I couldn't conceive of anything but being cancer free. I refused to say, "I have breast cancer."

I knew to speak healing as though I had already received it so I did. Scripture confirms that if we operate in the power of faith without doubt and simply be selective in our words, we shall receive what we ask: "Have Faith in God. I tell you the truth, if anyone of you says to this mountain, Go throw yourself into the sea, and does not doubt in his heart but believes that what he says will happen, it will be done for him. Therefore, I tell you whatever you ask for in prayer, and believe that you have received it and it will be yours (Mark 11:22-24). I still struggled with feelings of hurt and confusion, but I tell you, I daily spoke out loud, "I am cancer free. God has already healed me," and I never doubted it!

A week passed and Gary and I went to Dr. Mann's to discuss the biopsy results and treatment options. Having Gary with me was comforting; he was my extra ears and eyes in case I missed anything critical. I strongly encourage taking a partner with you to the doctor particularly when the news may be severe. I don't care how tough you are—a partner can help you recall what was said and is apt to listen with an objective and attentive ear because you may well be selective in your hearing.

Dr. Mann called my diagnosis Ductal Carcinoma In Situ (DCIS)—cancer cells inside the milk ducts, sometimes referred to as pre-cancer. He said this type was good news. He told us the cancer was in the best possible place, localized in one breast only, contained, and slow to spread. He explained that cancer is "staged," using a classification system that is based on tumor size, number of lymph nodes involved, and any spread to other organs. All the information is combined into the stage numbers 0-4 (best to worst). In my case, the disease was at Stage 0. Jump up and shout! This was excellent news!

But then came the bad news! He said I needed to have a mastectomy. A WHAT?!?! A Mastectomy?!?!?! Remove my breast?!?!?!?! No way!!! Those little white lint-looking specs on the mammogram couldn't be that harmful! There had to be other options!

Dr. Mann repeated that having a mastectomy was the best treatment option for an excellent prognosis. A lumpectomy was not recommended because I had no lump and the cancer was disseminated throughout the milk ducts. In my case, it would be difficult for the doctors to precisely excise only the infected ducts. Radiation wouldn't benefit me for the same reason; there would be no way to target a specific area. Chemotherapy at that point was not necessary because there was no evidence the cancer had spread. (I don't know what I expected my treatment would be, but I knew for sure a mastectomy wasn't it!) I sat on the examining table trying to process it all. I looked at Gary and then away to see if I could find God anywhere in the room.

The doctor kept talking, saying I could have a mastectomy, reconstruct the breast if I wanted to, and move on with my life normally. Reconstruction meant creating a new breast by way of plastic surgery and introduced a whole other set of options I didn't have the capacity to absorb at that moment. He kept asking and asking, "Do you understand what I'm saying to you, Mrs. Burgess? Do you understand?"

All I could do was nod yes, but I was starting to get angry. Dr. Mann sounded as if a mastectomy was a simple solution and that I should accept it just as simply! I didn't like his tone; it made me feel like I had to give him an answer right away. I suddenly felt rushed and pushed! How could he expect me to make such an important decision without giving me ample time to think? I was furious! Just cut it off and move on with my life? I didn't think so! (I found myself wondering if Dr. Mann would have been so matter of fact had the tables been turned and we'd been discussing testicular cancer. Would it have been easier for him to understand?)

My breasts were important to me! Aside from the fact I fed both my babies from them, I valued them for their physical appearance and how they completed my shapely figure. I valued the sexuality and femininity they represented. My breasts belonged to me. They were mine since birth—a set—how was I supposed to understand having one of them removed?

In retrospect, I realize I was in first-reaction-shock-mode and my sensitivity was over the top. I'm sure Dr. Mann is really an excellent surgeon, but he didn't meet my needs.

We left Dr. Mann's office and went directly to meet with an oncologist (cancer doctor). Gary and I twiddled our thumbs in the examining room until Dr. Hope arrived.

He was tall, dark, and handsome and had a very soothing voice and gentle bedside manner. His assistant drew my blood, he examined me, and then he explained his part in my treatment plan.

Let me say that doctors are funny—not humorous—but peculiar in their communication when they talk amongst each other and when they don't want to give you all the bad news at one time. Dr. Hope said his role was to determine whether I would need radiation, chemotherapy, or any other treatment after the surgery.

Surgery? WHO SAID I WAS HAVING SURGERY? What an assumption! I was only twenty minutes out of Dr. Mann's office and definitely hadn't agreed to any surgery! I appreciated this doctor's gentle touch, but I really wanted a second opinion.

I asked Dr. Hope if he knew Dr. Love, the female general surgeon I had originally tried to see. When he said that he did, I asked if he knew how I could possibly get an appointment with her.

"I will call her and see if she'll see you tomorrow if you'd like," he said. Needless to say, I liked!

That afternoon, while Gary and I were having lunch, I received a call from Dr. Love. We hadn't spoken for more than a minute before she calmly asked me when and where I was having my surgery. There was that word again! I told her that I hadn't decided to have surgery, much less scheduled its time and place, and she interrupted me to say, "Delores, from this point on you must stay focused and believe that you are going to be just fine. You will be all right, hands down!" She told me she would be happy to see Gary and me in her downtown office the next day!

Thank You, Jesus!

Chapter 3
Telling My Babies – More Pain

By 6:00 that evening, I was physically, emotionally, and spiritually whipped. In one day, I had spoken, either in person or by telephone, with three different doctors, but I still needed answers.

It was Wednesday, Bible Study night, and I was scheduled to sing at my church's (Voices of Faith) Leadership Conference on Thursday. I was too distracted for either. On the way home, Gary and I called the church to give my pastor the news and to tell him that I would not be singing at the conference the next day. One of our elders answered the phone and I tried to tell her the reason for my call but I broke down in tears before I could speak. Gary had to take the phone and finish the conversation for me.

Pastor called me back and I reiterated to him that I had been diagnosed with breast cancer and had a favored appointment to see Dr. Love, who was said to be one of the best, if not *the* best, breast cancer surgeon in the country.

"What does that have to do with your singing?" he asked.

WHAT????? If I could faint on demand I would have.

"A whole lot in my opinion!" I retorted. I needed to keep this appointment. He couldn't possibly understand!

He told me this was not the time to run and hide and that I should not try to deal with my problem alone and behind closed doors. I assured him that I wasn't hiding. I had a serious issue that demanded immediate medical attention and I had been shown favor to see Dr. Love.

He reminded me, as my spiritual father, that it was his job to push me. Then he asked if I would come and let him, and at least the elders, pray and lay hands over me. I told him that I would. Then he closed our conversation with prayer.

Now I had no choice but to go ahead and tell the girls. What an emotional hurdle it was to go inside and face them with this kind of news! After finishing my conversation with the pastor, I sat, for a moment, inside the garage. Again, I had to pull myself together so I could be strong for my babies.

Gary and I gathered the girls in our family room. They both looked at us as if we had done a poor job at keeping a secret from them. They had known for weeks that something was going on. Their faces were so sweet and I thanked God they were good and faithful girls and that they knew of Him.

As soon as I said the "C" word, the tears fell! It hurt tons to have to tell them. It wasn't fair…moms shouldn't have to impose undue burden and stress upon their children…not like this! But no matter. They needed to know.

I explained my diagnosis, the treatment option as I knew it, and the option to immediately reconstruct after surgery…if I chose to have surgery. I was explicit and honest with my girls about the diagnosis because it was their right to be properly informed. They were now at risk of getting breast cancer themselves. Plus, if I ended up having a mastectomy, I didn't want my surgery to go down in history as some "hush-hush watered down no-name female trouble." (Say "Amen" if you know what I'm talking about!)

Tiffany, who was fifteen at the time, listened intently. Camaren, my eleven year old, cried. She was all for the possibility of surgery and reconstruction because she did not want to see me with one breast on one side and none on the other. For the record, neither did I. Tiff didn't like the idea of an implant. She was aware of the associated dangers. Collectively, we decided that if I had the mastectomy, the TRAM Flap Reconstruction was our best option. This type of reconstructive surgery meant the plastic surgeon would take fatty tissue from my lower abdominal pouch, and use it to make a new breast. (This way I wouldn't need a breast implant and would get a more natural looking and feeling breast replacement, plus a tummy tuck to boot!)

Overall the girls took the news well! I teased them, saying that after my tummy tuck, I would be "finer" than both of them when it was all over!

We went to church as I had promised. Through hopeful tears, I shared the news with my church family. Sharing it meant hundreds more people were impacted by the diagnosis.

It felt good to be surrounded by all the love and support. We cried, rejoiced, declared healing, and blessed God with words of praise for his marvelous healing power. Massive prayer ascended from the house that night. Pastor laid hands on my head, his wife on my breast, our Minister of Music on my feet, and others on my head, back, waist, and stomach. All of the people at Voices of Faith that night exemplified the faith, hope, and love of one body sharing in the suffering of one of its members. I'm sure God was pleased!

Chapter 4
Peculiar Preparation and Perfect Arrangement

That night when I got home from church I replayed the entire day in my head. I concluded this was the most difficult day of my life. How could such a little person handle something this big? My five-foot, 115-pound frame didn't have wide enough shoulders to carry this load! I was overwhelmed, but before the night was over, I would be reminded that no Christian ever walks alone.

I retreated to the sunroom, my favorite room of the house, and listened for something to click in my head and make sense. The phone rang and it was my mentor and friend Clara Walton, President of Sisters Network, Atlanta Chapter (SNAC) and an eight year breast cancer survivor.

Yes, that's correct—breast cancer survivor! Clara was floored at hearing my news. She said she would never have thought, in a million years, that I would be relating to her from a patient standpoint. (Neither would I.) She gave me some really good advice and made me aware of several things I needed to consider.

She told me to be involved with my care and treatment plan and not to give the doctors total control—to push if I needed to and demand if I felt I should! I really appreciated her concern and wisdom.

You're probably wondering how I got connected to a breast cancer survivor so quickly. As a matter of fact, I rank my meeting Clara the most compelling aspect of my testimony. Let me first say, though, that after the phone call with Clara, things *did* begin to click and make sense, just as I had hoped.

I came to know Clara Walton and SNAC—an affiliate of the only national breast cancer organization run by African-American survivors—in September of 2002, an entire year before my diagnosis. I partnered with them (reluctantly, I might add), singing at one of their outreach events as a favor to my good friend Vickie, a breast cancer supporter who lost her aunt to the disease at the age of thirty-eight.

I wasn't looking to take on another "cause" as my focus and energy were directed to HIV/AIDS, the elderly, the poor and the youth. But I ultimately yielded to the overwhelming compassion I felt for Vickie, her aunt, and the many women who benefit from the inspiration SNAC has to offer. I agreed to do that one engagement and fell in love with the organization. The women of Sisters Network Atlanta labored out of love and provided the necessary function of promoting awareness among African-American women in the community! That single event charged me to become their honorary "songstress" and an associate member of the organization.

I began singing at their monthly meetings and other events as well as wholeheartedly promoting their mission. I made their brochures available at my singing events and referred people to them whenever the opportunity arose. I learned a lot about "being a survivor" and being involved in the support of breast cancer patients and their families. Most importantly, my interaction with SNAC reminded me of my own responsibility to perform breast self exams, get my mammograms on time, and to encourage others and make them aware of the same.

I never once correlated my involvement with SNAC with a possibility of ever having breast cancer myself. But

God had divinely placed me in the middle of a breast cancer survivor organization an entire year before I, myself, would be diagnosed with the illness.

Isaiah 46:9-10 says "Remember the former things, those of long ago; I am God and there is no other; I am God and there is none like me, I make known the end from the beginning"...WOW! My end was revealed in the beginning. It was confirmed a year before that I would survive!

Joy erupted underneath the layers of my deadened senses! God was definitely due glory and praise for His undeniable provision made exclusively for me in preparation for this journey. Not only had he placed me in SNAC, but He reminded me that he had blessed us with medical insurance only two months before the mammogram. We had been without health insurance for about six months after Gary's full-time employment was impacted by 9/11. We had considered a few plans but they were too expensive for us at the time.

A young gentleman showed up at our office selling independent health insurance plans for small businesses and entrepreneurs. He represented a major company—one that we had already considered and ruled out as an option. This young man was so certain we would qualify and could afford the plan that he convinced us to complete the application in spite of our apprehension over pre-existing conditions and our ability to pay the premium. In fewer than thirty days we were approved and God was evidently putting His "super" with our "natural" to get those monthly premiums paid.

And on top of it all, the insurance plan was such a good one that I didn't have to worry about selecting doctors from a preferred list because it allowed me to see any physician or specialist of my choice. Who but God knew what I needed?!!!

I reverenced Him, also, for the timeliness of the overwhelming urge I felt to have the mammogram in the first place. I had just celebrated my forty-first birthday and was completely amazed at how determined I was to have the mammogram. I was equally amazed at how I was not so compelled the year before.

And then there was the fact that before I had the biopsy, God had sent my friend LaNedra to tell me to check my breast. Gave it to her in a dream! She had no idea what I was dealing with when she declared that she heard God's voice clearly say, "TELL HER TO CHECK HER BREAST…TELL HER!"

When she shared this with me—two weeks before the biopsy—you could have picked my chin up from the floor! I was flabbergasted, but never admitted a thing! LaNedra stood mighty in the Lord, a prophetess by appointment, but because I hadn't been diagnosed at that time, I frankly refused to acknowledge her dream as a word of prophesy for me. She even suggested that I should have a mammogram!! All I could say was, "Maybe so."

My husband, Gary did, however, recognize the holy hand of God and was happy He sent LaNedra, a trusted friend, to give me a fair and peaceful warning. What a mighty God we serve!

All of these peculiar, precious deeds reminded me that God had my back! Without a doubt He knew exactly what I needed—when, where, and how I needed it.

Chapter 5
Faith, Faith, And More Faith

The following day, November 6, I had the face-to-face visit with Dr. Love. Gary and I arrived at 5:00 pm and there were four women ahead of me, one of whom had been there since 3:15 pm. I couldn't believe she had been waiting that long—it was obvious the doctor was running way behind. If ever there was a time to be patient, this was it!

Gary decided to find something to eat. I completed the necessary paperwork and prepared for the wait. I was sorry about reneging on singing at the conference that night but I wanted this appointment—I NEEDED this appointment. Finally, after 2 ½ hours, Dr. Love called us back. Let me just say now that the old adage is true. Everything good is worth waiting for.

Despite the lateness of the hour, Dr. Love spent more than two hours with us. Her staff went home one by one but she never showed any urgency about leaving herself. This lady was knowledgeable, thorough, easy to talk to, non-intimidating, smooth, straight to the point, and very patient. We asked question after question and she answered and explained everything.

After quite a while, she said, looking at me directly, "Delores, you are going to have to warm up to the fact that a mastectomy, though it seems to be an overly aggressive treatment, is your best option."

"Short of a miracle," I responded. I still wasn't ready to give in to the possibility.

She gave us greater insight regarding the options associated with breast reconstruction. She told me not to base my decision on internet information and photographs because the reality was quite different. She suggested I talk with some of her patients who had experienced it and take a look at their scars. I thought, WOW, who in the world would show me her breast, much less her surgical scars? This doctor was too much!

Dr. Love assured me that she was not a fan of scars and that she would take care not to make any unnecessary incisions. She understood clearly the traumatic effect a marred breast could have on the female self-esteem. We discussed all the options including saline (salt water) implants and breast prostheses (artificial substitutes).

I was about to collapse from information overload, but my brain kept signaling me not to worry. None of this talk would matter in a few days anyway because God was going to heal me without surgery! Gary must have been thinking the same thing because out of the blue, he suggested we do another biopsy, just to get another opinion. Dr. Love adamantly disagreed – but said she certainly could not stop us if we chose to move forward. She explained that she thought it would put us through unnecessary agony and stress.

No doubt we were stressed, but we were desperate to prove the diagnosis wrong. That would be so much better than my submitting to a surgery that would mutilate and debilitate me. We were bound in our faith and felt covered by the healing blood of Jesus Christ. We were banking on a miracle!

Dr. Love wrapped up all the medical and technical details and we began to talk more on a personal level. She advised us to do our homework and due diligence before making a final decision. She gave us the green light to enjoy

Thanksgiving but cautioned us not to linger beyond that. We got ready to leave (it was after 9:30 pm) and I was prompted to ask the doctor when she found time to rest.

"All I need is four hours and I'm good to go!" she said, declaring that she is gifted to do exactly what she does. Considering her spirit, the sacrifice of her time, and the professional expertise she displayed, I believe it to be so. She is one of God's miracle instruments, one who has the special gift to carry on His healing ministry and powerful works on earth! And God had assigned this awesome woman to me!

Let me say quickly that accepting all of this was no easy task for me. I had to minister over and over to myself to keep from falling in my faith. Some days I stood firm and other days I felt as though I was simply going through the motions. The *idea* of having faith was not enough.

Until I spoke with Dr. Love, I didn't begin to realize my trust in God was based only on a miracle of my choosing. To this point, I believed in only one way out—my way. I hadn't submitted to trust Him to supply every applicable means of healing available to me. Human Delores absolutely, unequivocally, did not want to have surgery, but waiting—even for a miracle—would yield me nothing. I needed to act and participate in the process. And participating meant activating mountain-moving faith with no preferences or limitations on the size of the mountain or what it would take to make it move.

God's plan always calls for the best. His presenting Dr. Love to me was confirmation that she was His best for me. After receiving this revelation, I submitted my total trust to God, and He immediately sent confirming witnesses, former patients, women from my church, individuals on the street, and folk from the health community to tell me of their experiences with Dr. Love. Every one of them told me I didn't have anything to worry about!

Mind you, to this point, this journey had been traveled with God seemingly at a distance and me plunging my way alone. I hope you can understand that I wasn't feeling any closer to God than I was the moon, but my thoughts were stuck on Him reminding and convicting me that He most certainly was there. This mental transformation centered my focus and dependence strictly on Him, and I discovered that the intimacy and closeness I desired and prayed for were not physical, but spiritual. Although the effects of the cancer would be felt physically, it would give me a greater opportunity to experience God spiritually. The bigger the problem, the greater the experience! I was beginning to live what I had known in my mind was the true meaning of trust:

* Trusting God means that we don't get to define the way in which our prayers are answered. God knows the way "out" and we don't. We often fail to recognize that our prayers have been answered until after the fact. Dr. Love would be one of those answers, and so would the breast cancer itself.

* Trust is not always a warm feeling. It is a spiritual event of surrender in the midst of painful circumstances we often try to control, but can't. It is the awareness that God's plan is best and the belief that He will act in the way that is best for us.

* It is pain, physical and emotional, that often jerks us back to an attitude of dependence on

God. It is easy, when things are going according to our plans, to focus our eyes on other things. God never promised us immunity from suffering—he promised us deliverance.

WOW! Three more revelations had come my way. I started digging and doing more research on breast cancer, ductal carcinoma in situ, stages of disease, mastectomies, lumpectomies, breast reconstruction, radiation, chemotherapy, alternative treatment options, and anything else I could find that might help me.

I would rather have discovered that I was different and the cancer inside me was not as bad as they thought, but all the medical information I read confirmed and re-confirmed the recommendations of all the doctors. (I'm not saying my findings made all of them right.) It just gave me an advantage in making an informed decision. Through all the reading and researching, I established a knowledge-based understanding of my diagnosis and some of the best known and most successful ways to treat it. Knowledge is Power!

Chapter 6
Telling My Family and Close Friend

It was time to tell the rest of my family…and my dear friend, Vickie. I drove to Chattanooga to tell my mother and stepfather in person. I knew I couldn't tell my mother over the phone. She needed to see that I looked healthy, was upbeat, and was as bright and positive as I usually am.

At first, she didn't quite grasp the certainty of it all. In shock, she asked a few probing questions like, "Are they sure it's cancer?" and "Do you have to have the surgery?" I felt her pain. It cut right down the middle of my chest but instead of crying, I squared my shoulders and lovingly gave it to her straight.

"There's no need for you to worry. My breast is offending me and I'm having the offense removed. I am confident in my faith, my medical team, and my treatment decisions. I am not afraid and I will be fine. God is going to take care of me." I left her no room to question me or to be left in denial. She looked at me with fear and sadness in her eyes.

Given some time, I knew she would send up a mother's prayer for me, and for her own peace of mind. She rubbed her chin, as she usually does when she's in deep thought, and finally said, "Okay."

I followed suit with my dad and my siblings, Rickie, Roger, Darryl, and Pat (sister). I left each of them with a request to pray for me and to believe God for my healing. I also made my sister and mother aware that they, too, were at risk and encouraged them to stay current with their annual exams and mammograms.

Vickie was like a sister to me, too, so telling her was just as emotional as telling the rest of the family. She was the booking manager for the ministry so we talked everyday. I hadn't given her any clue as to what was going on until the day I shared the news with her. Of course, she wrestled with the impact of this disease striking so close to home a second time.

Friends are so important at times like these yet sometimes they don't know quite what to say or do. You may be called on to be such a friend. If so, I hope you are blessed by her words and enabled by her actions. They meant a lot to me, so I want to share them with you here.

…WHAT!!! Oh my God! Did she just say what I thought she said? Pain began to spread over my entire body; I felt as if my heart had been punctured! How could this be? My daughter and I'd just enjoyed a wonderful weekend with Delores and her family. She didn't look like she had breast cancer, she didn't act like it, nor did she sound like it.

My mind frantically raced back to 1988, the year that my Aunt Viola died from breast cancer at thirty-eight years of age. She also was a Christian, had a successful career and was married with young children; her life was parallel to Delores'. I could not help but to wonder if Delores would succumb to the same fate. By now, I was overcome with fear. I began to grieve and re-live the familiar emotions of denial, helplessness, sorrow, anger, and hurt. Throughout the night, I petitioned God on Delores behalf and I cried until the following morning. It was then God gave me peace and what I perceived to be assurance that Delores was going to survive, although she was going to have to endure tremendous pain and suffering before she would be healed.

I realized this was no time for a pity party. Delores needed positive support from her family and friends. She needed to be surrounded with prayer warriors and fighters, those who possessed strength, courage, and faith. Those who would be willing to do whatever they could to make this journey more bearable for her. It was time to fight, to join in the battle against this highly feared and loathsome disease. How could I make a difference and truly be there for my sister, my friend? First, I had to become educated about breast cancer, the diagnosis, treatment options, and the recovery process. It was essential that I understood as much as possible about the disease so that I would be prepared to discuss it intelligently, contribute and give feedback as needed. Secondly, I had to be willing to assist with any practical needs, such as picking up the children, cleaning the house, cooking, and running errands. Thirdly, I had to be available to do whatever Delores wanted to do, whether it was going to the mall or just sitting in silence.

Delores actually made those things easy for all of us. She began to champion her own cause. Faith and bravery adorned her. From the beginning she claimed the victory and she battled faithfully and courageously every step of the way. Mentally she never acknowledged that the cancer was hers. Sure, it had invaded her body, but she would not own it, she would not allow it to stay! Her every action seemed focused on eradication, healing, and restoration.

Chapter 7
Don't Go Thinking I'm Crazy!

Gary, my girls, Vickie, family, my pastor and church family, Lanedra, her church family, everybody it seemed, was praying for me and pronouncing my total and complete healing. Prayer is Powerful!

I was enjoying my transformation and parading around in the bliss of victory. I had developed a new walk— a swagger, as my pastor says. I felt liberated! Healed! Yes, I went from educated and empowered to healed! So healed, in fact, that I began to waver on my commitment to surgery. I wasn't about to let them cut on me if I was already healed! I needed to go back for another mammogram and get proof! (Don't go thinking I'm crazy, now. I needed to check one last time…I had to!)

So, on Nov. 11, I skipped into Dr. Love's office to have that mammogram. While the technician was setting up, she asked, "When was your last mammogram?"

When I answered that I had had one in September, she was stunned, and asked why I was having another one so soon. I politely told her that it was because I wanted to.

She asked if Dr. Love knew I was there and if I was planning on seeing her, and then informed me that my insurance would only pay for one mammogram per year.

Why did she care? It wasn't her bill. I didn't know if Dr. Love knew I was there, I didn't know if she was going to see me or not, and I wasn't concerned about my insurance not paying…I REALLY DIDN'T CARE! I wanted another mammogram!

The tech left and the next thing I knew, Dr. Love had whisked into the room.

"Delores, what are you doing in here?" she asked.

"I'm getting a second mammogram. I want to check for God's glory…see if the cancer's still there."

She swelled up and looked me dead in the eyes. "This is crazy…I don't believe it. Do you really want this? Do you *really* want this?"

"Yes, I do."

"Why?"

"Because we have been in constant prayer and I want to make sure."

Dr. Love was taken aback. "Look," she said, "When God gives us something, he wants us to go through with it."

Adamant, I asked, "Do you believe in the power of prayer?"

"Yes I do," she answered, "but in this case, your having another mammogram won't tell me anything different."

"The first one did. Why not this one?" I was frustrated and couldn't understand her resistance. I asked if she had ever seen a case where "it" was there the first time and gone the next. She looked at me in disbelief and exclaimed, "Not with cancer!"

My eyes went light bulb size and I was frozen in shock. All I could say was "Really?"

She replied with an emphatic yes.

"In what cases have you seen whatever is on the mammogram go away?" I asked.

She responded that she had seen mammograms change with cysts, fibrosis, and a couple of other things that I didn't remember because, frankly, I stopped listening. I didn't want to believe her anyway…I really didn't. I told her this was something I needed to do, that it was part of my due diligence and I needed a second look for my own peace of mind before moving forward with surgery.

Human nature had gotten the best of me. I never mentioned it, but the thought of losing my breast was haunting me; I was already grieving. If there was any chance for me to save my breast, and if God had changed His will in response to the intervening prayers, I wanted to claim my miracle!

Dr. Love was concerned for me; she thought I was in big-time denial! I might have been to a point, but I wasn't avoiding treatment. After all, I wanted a second look! She couldn't convince me to change my mind, so she told the technician to go ahead and do it!

After the mammogram, Gary and I sat silently in the office waiting for the results. When she entered the room this time, Dr. Love immediately quizzed me, trying to get a fix on my psychological and emotional state. She explained that she thought I was in denial and that she did not want me to "go there" and not take care of my problem. I assured her that I was not in denial, and was fully prepared to take the next step if the results were the same. I told her that I was ready! I was just not going to spend the rest of my life wondering if I made the wrong decision and missed out on the miracle God had in store for me.

Please let me interject that true denial is a serious and unhealthy place to be. Many people suffer with cancer and other issues because they are unwilling to believe and especially, to acknowledge their conditions or situations. They reject the gift of doctors purposed to care for them here on earth.

Dr. Love believes wholeheartedly in interactive medicine and applauded my desire to be involved in my treatment and wanted me to be comfortable and secure in the decisions I made. She also clearly respected my faith. But she made it very clear that, as a scientist, she respected cancer, too. In her many years in practice she has seen the classic signs of denial. Her persistence to push me into reality came from having seen many women suffer and die from cancer unnecessarily.

As I'm sure you know, she was right about the mammogram. The results were exactly the same as before—I didn't get my version of a miracle that day. Gary cried as if we were hearing the news for the first time. He had counted on taking me home cancer free. Instead, he would have to trust God that he would do so at a later date.

The time had come to decide once and for all. I told Dr. Love, "Let's do the surgery!"

Chapter 8
My Mastectomy and God's Reconstruction

Dr. Love would perform a "skin-sparing" mastectomy, a procedure in which breast tissue is "scooped out," leaving the outer skin intact. Because milk ducts end in the nipple, she would also remove both the nipple and areola to minimize the risk of leaving behind any diseased cells.

For the immediate breast reconstruction, she referred me to Dr. Faith, a plastic surgeon who was a master with the TRAM FLAP procedure. He would do "his thing" after she finished the mastectomy. Together they were humbly known amongst their peers as "The A-Team!"

Gary and I went to see Dr. Faith right away. He, also handsome, was pleasant, patient, enthusiastic, and very spiritual. There was nothing about him I didn't like... thank God! He explained the process of reconstruction in as many details as we could comprehend, drawing pictures and simplifying seven-syllable terms.

He thought I was perfect for the TRAM FLAP procedure because I was small (in weight), healthy, and had good skin. He showed so much excitement that Gary and I couldn't help but be excited with him. We left his office feeling at peace, secure that we were in good and faithful hands. God had assigned another one of his healing instruments to me.

My team was set. The surgery was scheduled for December 10th (less than 2 weeks away). Having made the decision to go forward, my only concern now was surviving the operation itself. I believed I would be a cancer survivor but I also wanted to wake up, in my right mind, fully functional!

I began to prepare my home for my absence and long term recovery. Christmas was coming and I acted like a mama bird nesting for the season—cleaning, purging, and organizing. I was determined for my girls to have a good Christmas in spite of all the attention my breast was getting. I decorated the house, stocked up on groceries, and finished my Christmas shopping.

Some days were weird, because at times I felt as if I was preparing for my death. My eyes would well with tears and I would wince at the quick vision of my body lying in a casket. The sadness of losing my breast crept in and out, too, but I never missed a beat. I kept right on claiming victory and praising God as if it had already come!

On really difficult days, I found peace in hearing God say, "Have you tried, my good and faithful servant, Delores?" I praised Him for seeing a sustaining character in me. I, like Job, would come through the fire like pure gold (Job 23:10).

At my pre-op visit, Gary and I were sitting in the waiting room when the lady called me back, and as always, I asked Gary to come with me. She stopped us at the door and said, "I'd rather have Mrs. Burgess only."

I thought, Hmmm, that's different. I'm only giving blood and a pre-op interview and my husband can't be in the room? So I asked politely, "He can't come with me?"

"Well," she said, "the room is small and we prefer to have the patient only because sometimes family members get in the way, especially if I have to do an EKG."

What? After entering the room I assessed it was plenty big enough for him to join me! I didn't understand. My husband had accompanied me to every appointment and she was giving me this foolishness!

As if I needed more stress in my life, I actually got into an argument with her over the size of the room and the number of people it would hold. I could only guess that she must have had a bad experience prior to my coming and was taking her frustrations out on us.

I insisted Gary be present. After a moment, she reluctantly went to get him and made a point of telling him I had insisted. Something changed, though, because when she returned with Gary her demeanor was more pleasant. She asked my occupation and appeared to be impressed that I was a gospel singer in full-time ministry. In the end, we had a great interview and the technician apologized sincerely for upsetting me. Before we left, she gave us both a hug.

Wednesday, December 10th showed up as expected. I was up late the night before but fortunately rested very well, as I had to be at the hospital at 6:30 a.m.

I got up, prayed, and prepared for the imminent departure. The whole family was stirring in the house; it was a school day. My girls opted to come with us instead of going to school. They wanted to be there when I woke up, and I was thrilled.

My mom and Vickie had come down from Chattanooga. I was overjoyed that God had enabled my mother to come. She is a dialysis patient and though I didn't want to put any more stress on her, she was determined to be there for her "baby girl" And she was. (God even worked it out so she wouldn't miss her dialysis treatment.)

We formed a circle and prayed. I petitioned God on their behalf and I made my own requests known. I looked around at my beautiful home and vowed I would be back.

Gary and I rode together in our van. As we drove, we listened to gospel music; the ride was calm and peaceful, but by the time we reached the downtown area, he and I were both silently crying. I could see tears glistening on his dark-skinned face and he could hear the sniffles as I praised God with my voice. The song "God Can," by my mentor and friend, Dottie Peoples, was ministering to our souls, reminding us that JESUS, HE WILL FIX IT!

As I praised God, I looked up to the heavens and in the distant sky I could see the top floors of the hospital. I took a deep breath and cried even more, but as we arrived I composed myself and dried my face. I wanted to be strong for my girls and I was ready for it to be over.

It was hard to say "bye" to my loved ones even for only a few hours. I hugged my girls with a love that crushed my already broken heart. They were to perform at a dance recital in a day or so and for the first time, I wouldn't be backstage waiting to help them change or to give moral support. (My girls are excellent dancers and as I fought back the tears, I told them to "knock 'em dead, make me proud, and don't worry about me" and that I would see them later.)

After I was prepped for surgery, I was allowed to have visitors. My mom got a little squeamish looking at the surgical lines drawn on my breast and stomach. Wanda, my friend and fellow gospel artist, came back, to my surprise. Joyce, another dear friend, was also there. I've since thought that they must really love me to have gotten up that early in the morning to come to the hospital in support of me and my family.

Finally, Gary, Vickie and I waited for the doctors to come and get me for surgery. We laughed and joked about everything. Dr. Love came first and then Dr. Faith, and he asked if we could pray. I was pleased as he humbled himself before the Lord and expressed his dependence on God to guide his hands, eyes, and mind. My CD, "Faith All Over It" would play while the surgeries were being performed. (For some stupid reason, I thought I would hear some of it, too…NOT! I was knocked out long before I entered the operating room.)

The surgery took about three and a half hours. I remember waking up and asking, "Am I alive?" I managed to clear my vision enough to see the blur of a nurse moving about and checking me. She was asking me questions and I was responding in between agonizing moans. I heard her yell to someone that I needed more pain reliever.

The next thing I remember was being rolled to my room. All my visitors were crammed into it. Sitting and standing, they were wall to wall, but I was so happy to see all of their faces.

From that point on nurses and technicians came in and out of my room for what seemed like every half hour. I was told I needed to keep the reconstructed breast warm and at a certain temperature for the first twenty-four hours. A cold spot in the breast would mean the blood was not flowing through the TRAM flap correctly and the involved tissue might not survive.

Torture ruled when I had to cough and do breathing exercises in that plastic breathing apparatus. It was down right gut wrenching but I did it anyway. I didn't want to get pneumonia.

The day after my surgery, I sat on the sofa for about thirty minutes. I was really out of it from the pain medication. I couldn't stand up straight. I had to bend at the waist due to the sixteen-inch incision that extended across my entire front (hip to hip). The pain was light years greater than a Caesarean (I had one with both daughters) and I needed lots of assistance. Thankfully, I was able to administer my own pain medication, though I sometimes slept too long without giving myself a dose and awakened in severe pain.

On day two, I walked the hospital corridor. It took a little while but my technician was patient and gentle with me. We laughed at my snail's pace.

I was extremely nauseated. Gary and Vickie placed cold compresses on my throat to curb it, but it only worked for a little while. I finally got medicine to help with the nausea. Because I was on a liquid diet, my stomach was empty except for the ice chips and water I had consumed.

I thought my skin had become super dry all of a sudden because I itched like crazy, but we learned that it was caused by the anesthesia. Vickie scratched and rubbed my arms and back, and applied lotion to soothe the itch while my mom lubricated my lips. (I told everybody before we left the house that it was mandatory that they all assume Vaseline® duty. Their orders were: DO NOT LET MY LIPS GET CHAPPED!)

Gary sacrified the most, though. He slept on the little hospital sofa convertible, not the most comfortable bed, and helped me attend to my drainage bulbs. Not one, not two, but three of these things extended from my body like alien arms (two from my stomach incision, one from the reconstructed breast). We had to measure, record, and drain the fluid and then clean the bulbs afterwards and Gary did it all. When I showered, he stood outside holding the bulbs for me. He always got wet, and I know his arms were tired from holding the bulbs at a height where they wouldn't pull at my body. He even washed the parts of me I couldn't reach. Bless his heart, my honey never complained or acted as if any of it was a burden.

Sunday finally came and it was time to go home. I was still "sick as a dog," and when I stood up to get in the wheelchair I threw up my lunch. OUCH!—it hurt—and it was gross!!! The car ride was no more pleasurable, but it felt good knowing my destination was home.

As I stood in the foyer, the memories of the morning we left for the hospital took me away into a sea of sadness. The house was just as I'd left it. I felt like I had been in a dream.

My eyes filled with water as I remembered how we had prepared for my coming home. Gary and I had set up the downstairs guest room as my recovery haven because we knew I wouldn't be able to climb the stairs. He had even moved the computer desk into the room so he could work and watch over me, and I could use it when I was ready. As I breathed the familiar air of home, I appreciated the memories and the tears. God had answered my prayers— every one of them and then some! I called it all a perfect arrangement, a masterful plan that delivered me.

I don't want you to miss the fact that God's ways are available to all of us. To receive and accept them, we have to be trusting of Him. There is nothing special about me that deserved or earned the favor of God. The Bible says He hears the cries of the righteous and heals the brokenhearted. It also says He is close to the brokenhearted and binds their wounds.

True. True. True. God kissed my pain and bound the pieces of my broken heart. I was home, and though I faced a long physical recovery ahead, my head, heart, spirit, and soul were all in one accord! The cancer was gone, and

I expected nothing short of a full and complete recovery. Glory, Glory, Hallelujah, His truth was marching on...

Chapter 9
Recovery - Loving Me

Pain, pain medication, sleep, moans, and groans. If it hurt, I felt it. I have to say, though, that Gary was an excellent caregiver. He never looked at me with anything but love and adoration. My man was still very much attracted to me and whether I had a new breast or no breast, his actions said it didn't matter as long as he still had me. I thanked God for his unconditional love and considered myself better than blessed to have him as my husband.

He made me three meals a day, kept my water bottles filled, and helped me change my bandages. Every time I looked at my body, he, too, wanted to see how my healing was coming along. Gary stayed by my side, carefully planning his comings and goings from the room as well as the house. The girls were out of school for the holidays and he made sure one of them was at my bedside when he had to leave the room. WHAT A MAN, WHAT A MAN, WHAT A MIGHTY GOOD MAN!

At home, the drainage bulbs were more of a nuisance. Though I wasn't going anywhere anytime soon, they were restricting. I had to sleep mostly on my back and if I didn't bandage the bulbs' tubing just right, it would hurt, hurt, hurt! Putting clothes on over the drains was a challenge and when I had visitors I tried to creatively disguise them under my pajamas. Showering, thank God, was not as much of a chore after I came up with the idea to fasten the bulbs to my shower curtain with safety pins. This freed my hands so I could bathe and do stretching exercises without having Gary stand outside the curtain getting wet. I was never more thrilled than when I got rid of those things!

I loved looking at my flat stomach; I had lost eight pounds altogether. The reconstructed breast, to my surprise, looked really good. (Actually it was beautiful!) I often chuckled at the complexity of using my belly fat to make a new breast and the process of moving the flap of fat up to my chest...unbelievable! I was sure I would have some unsightly deformity or permanent scarring but that wasn't the case at all. It was without blemish. Though there was no areola or nipple, I had a great match to the shape, size, and feel of my other breast and I was happy! The finishing touches to come didn't concern me at all. I knew they wouldn't be added until approximately twelve weeks after surgery. I praised God for the miracle because this "sista" was cancer-free and F-I-N-E!

Aside from my plans for life after surgery, recovery became boring once I was awake for long enough stretches to realize it. January 2004 rolled in and the girls were back in school; Gary was job-hunting. I couldn't sit up for very long and grew tired of lying down, but I was able to manage on my own.

It was winter, and I am definitely not a cold weather person, so I was in no hurry to indulge in any outdoor activities. However, by the end of January, I needed to breathe some fresh air. I wanted to walk and get a little exercise.

At this point, about six weeks after surgery, I was able to stand straighter and move around more...slowly. I started taking regular walks and eventually worked my way up to a slow paced jog at about ten weeks. Jogging felt good because it eased my aching stomach when muscle spasms, due to the surgery, were super-duper-intense. (I'm talking about muscle spasms that felt like long monstrous labor contractions! Whew!)

On March 17, I went back to Dr. Faith for the nipple reconstruction surgery. In lieu of a skin graft, I chose the nipple-sharing procedure, in which the top portion of the unaffected nipple is used to get a better match. I allowed Dr. Faith to liposuction my TRAM site and smooth out some of the lumpiness around the incision.

I hadn't expected it, but the surgery wiped me out! I came home from the hospital the same day nauseated, sickly, and terribly weak. No one forewarned me that I would experience such a setback. I was black, blue, and purple for at least two weeks; I was listless and lethargic and the pain was almost unbearable. A few days after surgery a severe pain erupted in my lower abdomen that was so horrific I couldn't put my feet flat on the floor to walk and had to tip-toe or crawl when I needed to move about. I guess my body wasn't ready for the added trauma or the effects of having anesthesia again so soon.

But, praise God, this too eventually passed and I began to feel better. Our bodies are amazingly resilient! My incisions were healing well and I loved my new body.

All I needed now was an areola tattoo. Hats off to the person who came up with tattooing the areola on a reconstructed breast! What a neat way to avoid surgical cuts and restore the natural look of the breast! We had fun mixing the colors to get the right hue. I was most excited about getting the tattoo because it meant that all of my bodily modifications would be completed by my birthday.

I had no problem looking in the mirror. As a matter of fact, I marveled at how symmetrical and physically correct I looked in a bra. I was glad that I had had the mastectomy and reconstructive surgery at the same time.

Going through reconstructive surgery is not for everybody, though. It is hard on the body and recovery from it is no joking matter. As you have read, it can take a long time to bounce back.

I, frankly, did not want the responsibility of putting in a prosthesis everyday. I feared, with my fast paced, on the go, spur of the moment, public lifestyle, I would one day forget to put it in before an appearance and not realize it until after I had seen the replay on television. I honestly feel immediate breast reconstruction may have saved me from an embarrassing but hilarious situation. I am glad I did it.

That, after all, is the point. It doesn't matter whether women go through reconstructive surgery, wear prostheses, or choose neither. Every woman faced with this decision should do what will ultimately make her feel best about the decision. We simply need to wear it and wear it well.

Beyond normal phantom pains, itching where I couldn't feel the scratch, and some numbness and soreness, I had no significant post-operative problems. My prognosis was EXCELLENT! Once again, I deluded myself a little, and assumed I would need no additional treatment.

I knew from my research that the probability of my needing chemotherapy was nil and had convinced myself that, alone, the mastectomy was an aggressive enough treatment to rid me of the cancer for life. My wishful thinking didn't change the fact that my doctors explained that any need for additional treatment following surgery would be determined based on the pathology of my breast tissue. (The bottom line was, of course, that I didn't want to make another treatment decision. I just wanted to be done.)

It was recommended that I take Tamoxifen (Nolvadex®). Commonly prescribed as an adjuvant, or secondary, treatment following a mastectomy in early stage breast cancer, Tamoxifen reduces the chance of cancer returning and helps prevent development of cancer cells in the other breast.

Dr. Hope explained that I had had cancer cells that respond to estrogen, making me what is known as "estrogen-receptor positive." Being pre-menopausal didn't help matters, either, because my body was still producing estrogen. Because estrogen promotes cancer cell growth, Tamoxifen works against the effects estrogen has on the growth of cancer cells.

I thoroughly researched the drug's benefits and risks before agreeing to take it. I found the typical descriptive and side effect information insightful, but some of the personal testimonials I came across were very alarming. Even so, I came to the conclusions that every person is different and it would do me no good to worry about being affected in a hundred different ways.

We decided that I would take the usual regimen of one pill per day for five years. And I was also offered four treatments of chemotherapy. Dr. Hope explained that the chemo would increase my chances of a non-recurrence by 2%. He went on to explain that some women want to take every possible measure, however small its effect, to reduce the chance of cancer's return.

I can certainly understand that reasoning but I elected not to pursue chemo. I was aware of the potential for harsh side effects and had done enough research to know that the Tamoxifen, in conjunction with the mastectomy, was probably sufficient in my case.

I told Dr. Hope I would ask God to "cover" me for that 2% and more. I am thankful that I had a choice. My regard is the highest for all individuals whose diseases require that they undergo chemotherapy. They deserve badges of honor.

Chapter 10
Back On The Front Lines

My doctors told me it would take at least a year for my body to return to normal. I spent a great portion of that time immersed in enough breast cancer literature to create an in-home library. I always knew I would be involved more heavily in the cause of breast cancer once I was back on my feet. By April 2004, I returned to the front lines with SNAC, educating and reaching out to people at various health fairs and events like the Tour de Georgia with Lance Armstrong. I enjoyed attending informational meetings and talking with people from every walk of life. There was a "big ole breast cancer world out there" with plenty of people giving of themselves to help cancer victims and I was called to be one of them!

My journey with breast cancer proved purposeful. Getting involved and making a difference—big or small—was crucial for me. Most every day I was in contact with someone either directly or indirectly affected by breast cancer. I was always saddened at the number of females who were not aware of how to do a breast self-exam or the fact that they should do one and why. (There exists an enormous need for breast health education, awareness, and self-empowerment.)

Being on the front lines also meant advocating and being informed about issues and developments related to the disease and having an assessment of the community and its needs. I found there were so many resources available to breast cancer patients if they knew only how and which resources to access. Survivor organizations, support groups, foundations, coalitions, health and educational programs, services, insurances, initiatives, workshops, ministries, legislature...all folded into the pie. In my position, I had a voice! If I couldn't do anything else, I could speak and act on behalf of those who unfortunately may not have an opportunity to speak for themselves.

Before I knew it, June, my favorite month of the year, was bringing in the sunshine! I was about to celebrate my forty-second birthday and six months of survivorship! In the midst of all the activity and a move into our new home, I transitioned into full time work at the American Cancer Society. Already a part of their Speakers Bureau, I went on board as a Recruitment Specialist for the Making Strides Against Breast Cancer Walk.

I was elected Vice President of SNAC and become a Trainer of Excellence for the "Reach Out and Learn" Initiative which provides breast and prostate cancer health education, inspirational support, and facts on community impact. As Vice President, I represented the organization at initiative meetings and focus groups conducted by projects under the National Black Leadership Initiative on Cancer II: Network Project (NBLIC II) at Morehouse School of Medicine.

One of the NBLIC projects—Men Against Breast Cancer—puts special emphasis on the crucial role of the husband/partner in caring for the woman he loves. I was fortunate enough to be able to offer my own experience and practical and professional knowledge as a part of the first focus group held in Atlanta. As a result of it, Gary agreed to participate in the all-male focus group and training and deemed the experience one of the most gratifying things he had ever participated in! He now assists MABC as needed.

From support to science and research, I was motivated for it all! Clara Walton graciously nominated me to be a Consumer Reviewer of research proposals, with her as my mentor, for the 2004 Department of Defense Breast Cancer Research Program in Washington, DC. A tremendous honor and privilege, I welcomed the opportunity to work with scientists in developing the best methods to prevent, treat, and cure breast cancer. My efforts qualified me to participate in the 2005 reviews.

Chapter 11
Blessed To Be A Witness

October 2004—Breast Cancer Awareness Month—rolled around and I was busy through the middle of November speaking, singing, inspiring and motivating! Aside from these events, I had accepted only a few light ministry engagements. I wasn't physically ready for much more.

My full time ministry had been on hold and in the days leading up to this time, I focused on regaining my vocal strength and patiently listening for God's direction as to where He wanted me to go.

Did I mention that on October 10, 2004, I had my annual mammogram? Yes, and I did it without hesitation. My results were NORMAL!!!! Hallelujah!!!! I was FREE of cancer and glad to be alive. I made sure God knew it, too!

The holidays seemed to slow things down a bit, which allowed me time to reflect on my fellowship with God. Whew! His grace and mercy had ushered me through another phenomenal year! My life was changed, never to be the same again! I was a new creature observing the intricacies of life with new eyes and a renewed mind. Things that had mattered in the past didn't anymore. Worry and stress were not instant coping mechanisms for me anymore. I appreciated the fresh air and the ability to breathe. My sights became set on purposeful things, simplicity, and peace!

God had delivered me to His bosom and I was enjoying an intimacy with Him there. I had come to know Him better and as a result I became a better person, wiser in spirit and stronger in character.

By the time I finished writing the first draft of this book, I had reached the end of my journey through the shadow of breast cancer. As always in His perfect timing, God spoke to me through my pastor and reminded me of my appointed duty. My voice—the God-given gift to sing—was very much intact and I had promised Him before any of this happened I would use my gift for Him forevermore. He assured me my gift would make room for me to do an even greater work for the breast cancer cause.

Now I see myself a complete package, divinely broken and restored for the good of others. By this, I mean God has blessed me with the ability to meet people where they are, a discerning and compassionate spirit compelled to reach out, knowledge and intellect to teach, a profound personal experience to relate, a motivational speaking ministry to encourage, and a soul-stirring musical therapy to soothe.

I love people and have made myself available to go wherever the need dictates. I use my relationships with churches, businesses, schools and community leaders to establish platforms to consistently push the mission of organizations like Sisters Network, Sisters by Choice, and The Witness Project.

The fact that African-American women are dying senselessly at alarming rates, primarily due to late stage diagnoses, keeps me determined to use every opportunity I'm afforded to shake women up and get them to realize the importance of education and early detection. I want us all to be empowered, by knowledge at least, to take responsibility for our bodies. I desire to assist women and men with dispelling the cultural myths, risky behaviors, superstitions, and fears that keep them from being proactive regarding their health.

One of the things I continue to appreciate about Dr Love is that she does whatever it takes to reach out to her patients. While I was at her office for a follow-up visit, she used me to speak to someone drowning in devastation. Whatever it took—a hug, my shoulder to cry on, or a look at my reconstructed breast—I was willing to help. It's moments like these that keep me humble. Just as Dr. Love declares she is gifted to do what she does, I believe I am, too. Praise God!

§

Well now, I've said it all. Thank you for reading Suspicion of Malignancy. I hope you've been inspired by my faith, encouraged by my journey, and motivated by my joy. You have the same opportunity to achieve victory and triumph in your situation as I did. The spirit does not discriminate and God does not lie, regardless of the varying degrees of difficulties, problems, and struggles we face. We win through the consequences of our choices (the spirit led ones)!

No matter how bad things may seem, you must consciously decide to act with your faith and not react with your flesh. Let's face it, some things just can't be dealt with in the flesh, and devastation by way of cancer is one of those things. God can handle any problem; let Him! Trust Him! You've just witnessed what He's done in my life. I cannot guarantee the same outcome, but I can guarantee that if you call on Him, He will provide you with all you need to face whatever adversity confronts you.

If you are so far down the road that you can't remember anything else I said in the book, remember this:

CHOOSE LIFE! CELEBRATE! LIVE!

APPENDIX

About Breast Cancer and Mammograms

Just the mere mention of the word "mammogram" makes a lot of the women I encounter very edgy—particularly those who have never had one. Some clutch their hands to their chests, or shall I say breasts, as if needing to shield their precious jewels from some horrific violation, or as if they are cringing from the unbearable pain they've heard is caused by a mammogram. Some nervously explain why they have never treated themselves to a mammogram, aiming to convince me that it really isn't necessary for them to have one since nobody in their family has ever been diagnosed with this type of cancer. Many respond under the influence of the misperception that they shouldn't go looking for something they don't want to find—while a great many, out of ignorance, innocently opt against having a mammogram because their philosophy on health is that they only go to a doctor if they're sick.

Of all the hundreds of women I've spoken to about breast cancer awareness and breast health I'm concerned most for the ones who have a family history and still go on silently and casually avoiding a mammogram. I guess they have decided that breast cancer, for them, is inevitable. They have lost grandmothers, mothers, aunts, and in some cases, combinations of all three to the disease and are resigned in their expectation that they, too, will develop the disease. Some of them tell me "I don't want to know!" When I hear this, I pray for the power of persuasion to be unleashed through me immediately.

No woman should be held hostage by the fate of her loved ones nor should she give up defending her own health and pay the awful price of being afraid, when a simple mammogram could very well save her life!

According to the American Cancer Society, breast cancer is the most common cancer among women. It is also the second leading cause of cancer deaths among African American woman, surpassed only by lung cancer. I wish I could twinkle my nose and magically change all of the perceptions and misguided reactions that some women have towards mammograms. It is my desire that every woman will gladly "step up to the plate" and handle her business with total grace and confidence!

Men be aware. You are not exempt. Don't let the chest fool you—men get breast cancer too! One in every 100 breast cancer cases is a man.

If you have a family history of breast cancer, you should definitely speak with your doctor about being screened, but all men are potentially at risk, and should do breast self-exams, checking for unusual lumps beneath the nipple. If a lump is found, get it checked immediately. Breast cancer is as curable in men as it is in women. But because breast cancer is unusual in men, it can easily go unnoticed and untreated, decreasing the odds of survival. (For more info visit www.menstuff.org.)

Please, whoever you are, take charge of your breast health by having regular mammograms, getting clinical breast exams, and performing breast self-exams. Empower yourself with the knowledge of early detection guidelines and uphold the assurance that although it's not perfect, a mammogram is the single most effective method for finding breast cancer early. It is the best defense!

It certainly was mine. Had I not gone for that routine mammogram I would never have known I was living with cancer. Finding it early afforded me the most effective treatment options and the highest chances for a total cure.

We need more positive outcomes like this! We need to celebrate more survivors! So, I'm saying to you what LaNedra said to me: CHECK YOUR BREASTS! If you are female, age 40 or older, and you have not had a mammogram, put this book down RIGHT NOW and call your physician to schedule one, and when you're done, pat yourself on the back. You will have made a wise and potentially life-saving choice! You have joined the ranks of women who are diligent and consistent with making sure their breasts are cared for and best guarded against breast cancer. Be sure to follow it through!

American Cancer Society: Cancer Facts & Figures for African Americans, 2003-2004

From 2003-2004, an estimated 20,000 newly diagnosed cases of breast cancer are expected to occur among African American women, and 5,700 of them are expected to die with the disease.*

American Cancer Society: Cancer Facts & Figures 2004.

Breast cancer is the most common cancer among African American women and the second leading cause of cancer deaths among this ethnic group, surpassed only by lung cancer. African American women five- year survival rate of breast cancer is 74%, compared to white women of 88%.**

From the Sisters Network Inc. Brochure

Sisters Network recommends the following steps for early detection:

* Monthly self breast exams starting at age 20.

* Clinical breast exam by trained medical professional every 2-3 years beginning at age 20 and annually at age 40

* Annual Mammogram screening for women age 35 (if your mother or sister has had breast cancer, you may need to get a mammogram earlier and more frequently).

Scriptures that held me up when…

…my imagination would run away with me; My thoughts became gory and gloomy; I thought I might die.

Casting down imaginations and any high thing that exhaulteth itself against the knowledge of God, bringing into captivity every thought to the obedience of Christ.
(2 Corinthians 10:5)

Indeed, in our hearts we felt the sentence of death. But this happened that we might not rely on ourselves but on God, who raises the dead. (2 Corinthians 1:9)

…I was scared, weak, powerless, and seemingly out of my mind.

For God has not given us a spirit of timidity (fear) but a spirit of power, of love, and self-discipline (sound mind).
(2 Timothy 1:7).

Therefore, my dear friends, as you have always obeyed not only in my presence, but now much more in my absence continue to work out your salvation with fear and trembling, for it is God who works in you to will and to act according to his good purpose. (Philippians 2:12-13)

…my heart was broken; I was hurt and devastated.

The Lord is close to the broken hearted and saves those who are crushed in spirit. (Psalm 34:18).

He heals the broken hearted and binds up their wounds.
(Psalm 147:3)

...I needed prayer; couldn't pray; wanted the multitude praying for me.

Is any one of you sick? He should call the elders of the church to pray over him and anoint him with oil in the name of the Lord. And the prayer offered in faith will make the sick person well; the Lord will raise him up. If he has sinned, he will be forgiven. Therefore confess your sins to each other and pray for each other so that you may be healed (James 5:14-15).

...I was doubtful; Couldn't see healing and wanted to believe but wasn't sure how to do it.

"Have Faith in God," Jesus answered. "I tell you the truth, if anyone of you says to this mountain, Go throw yourself into the sea, and does not doubt in his heart but believes that what he says will happen, it will be done for him. Therefore, I tell you whatever you ask for in prayer, and believe that you have received it and it will be yours." (Mark 11:22-24)

...I would lose my focus and felt cancer was too much for me to handle.

No temptation has seized you except what is common to man. And God is faithful; he will not let you be tempted beyond what you can bear. But if you are tempted, he will also provide a way out so you can stand up under it (I Corinthians 10:13).

...I forgot how God had cared for me thus far.

Remember the former things, those of long ago; I am God and there is no other; I am God and there is none like me, I make known the end from the beginning. (Isaiah 46:9-10)

…my fleshly emotions tried to control me; I couldn't see what God was doing.

Do not conform any longer to the patterns of this world, but be transformed by the renewing of your mind. Then you can test and approve of what God's will is – His good pleasing and perfect will. (Romans 12:2)

…I needed to be patient, find positive perspective, and see the purpose of my pain.

Not only so, but we also rejoice in our suffering, because we know that suffering produces perseverance; perseverance, character; and character, hope. And hope does not disappoint us, because God has poured out his love into our hearts by the Holy Spirit, whom he has given us. (Romans 5:3-5)

…I refused to give up!

Consider it pure joy, my brothers, whenever you face trials of many kinds because you know that the testing of your faith develops perseverance. Perseverance must finish its work so that you may be mature and complete, not lacking anything. If any of you lacks wisdom, he should ask God, who gives generously to all without finding fault, and it will be given to him. But when he asks, he must believe and not doubt, because he who doubts is like a wave of the sea blown and tossed by the wind. (James 1:2-6).

…I couldn't help but praise God for keeping me on this earth.

Give thanks to the Lord, call on his name; make known among the nations what he has done. Sing to him, sing praise to him, tell of all his wonderful acts, Glory in his holy name; Let the hearts of those who seek the Lord rejoice. Look to the Lord and his strength; seek his face always. Remember the wonders he has done, his miracles, and the judgments he pronounced. (I Chronicles 16:8-12)

Scripture for Salvation:

My friend, if my testimony has enlightened you yet you do not have a personal relationship with God, I want you to know that you can start one right now. All you have to do is willingly and sincerely pray out loud, if you can, and ask Jesus to come into your life:

Lord Jesus I know I am a sinner and need your forgiveness. I know you died on the cross for me. I now turn from my sins and ask You to forgive me. I now invite you into my heart and life. I now trust You as Savior and follow You as Lord. Thank You for saving me. Amen.

Read the scripture below. This is your confirmation that He will come at this very moment.

Every one who calls on the name of the Lord will be saved. (Romans 10:13)

Congratulations, Welcome To God's family!

Frequently Asked Questions

Wherever I go to speak about breast cancer, I am often asked questions about my experience. Though many of the answers were provided in the text of Suspicion of Malignancy, I have listed below the most frequently asked questions and my answers to those questions.

How old were you when you were diagnosed?
41.

How long have you been a survivor?
2 years.

Did you discover the cancer yourself?
No, via mammogram. My first!

Was it in both breasts?
No, just one.

Did you have a lump?
No. I didn't have any symptoms at all.

Was it caught early?
Yes!

Has anyone in your family had breast cancer?
No, not that I'm aware of.

Were you afraid?
Yes!

Did you cry?
Yes!

Did you feel alone?
Totally!

Were you angry?
More like furious!

When did you tell your husband and children?
My husband was informed immediately after every event. I told my children nothing until after the biopsy confirmed the malignancy.

Did you get a second opinion?
Yes.

How did you come to decide to have surgery?
My choices were limited and I knew I couldn't handle trying to make a drastic lifestyle change...or waiting. I had enough information to convince me.

Did you have to have chemo or radiation?
No.

Did you have a mastectomy?
Yes.

Did you reconstruct with implants?
No.

What type of reconstruction surgery did you have?
Tram Flap.

What the heck is a TRAM flap?
Plastic surgery that uses your lower abdominal fat and tissue to build a new breast. It stands for Transverse Rectus Abdominus Musculocutaneous Flap.

Was your husband supportive?
Yes. Very much so. I couldn't have asked for a better source of support.

Did he go to your doctor visits with you?
Yes. All of them prior to surgery and as needed afterwards.

After surgery did your husband look at or treat you any different?
No, he was very loving. Glad to have me alive and cancer free.

How long was your recovery?
I'm still recovering, but began feeling more like myself after about a year and a half.

How long after were you intimate with your husband?
Approximately four months.

Do you have any feeling in the reconstructed breast?
Yes, but only around the outer areas.

What does your reconstructed breast look like?
Very much like the other one, but slightly firmer.

Does it feel natural?
Yes, soft and warm to the touch. Still some numbness.

Are you embarrassed at being intimate with your husband?
Not at all.

Bibliography

Voluminous literature—books, pamphlets, and brochures—is often given women diagnosed with breast cancer. In my experience, some of the information can be extremely helpful. This bibliography lists the reading materials and internet websites I personally found helpful while going through the process, and while working on this book.

Disciples Study Bible, Holman Bible Publishers, 1988

The Holy Bible – New International Version, The International Bible Society, 1973, 1978, 1984

Dr. Susan Love's Breast Book, Susan M. Love, M.D. with Karen Lindsey—Third Edition, A Merloyd Lawrence Book, Perseus Publishing, Cambridge, Massachusetts, 2000

A Woman's Decision: Breast Care, Treatment, & Reconstruction, Karen Berger and John Bostwick III, 3rd ed. Quality Medical Publishing, Inc. St Louis, Missouri, 1999

The Purpose-Driven® Life, Rick Warren, Zondervan, Grand Rapids, Michigan, 2002

The American Cancer Society Brochures
www.cancer.org

The Sisters Network Celebrating Survivorship Brochure
www.SistersNetworkInc.org

www.breastcancer.org

The Susan G. Komen Breast Cancer Foundation
www.Komen.org

CURE–Cancer Updates, Research & Education Magazines

NOTES

NOTES

NOTES

NOTES

NOTES

To Book Delores Burgess for:

- Music Ministry
- Corporate Event Performances
- Inspirational Speaking
- Mistress of Ceremonies
- Speeches on Breast Health

Please call
770-469-4779
or
complete the booking form at
www.DeloresBurgess.com.

Most Requested Topics:

- Suspicion of Malignancy Testimony
- Victory In Motion
- Positive Perspective and Purpose
- Vision Beyond Bounds